Weight Loss and Nutrition

Health Media of America Editorial Board

i

Weight Loss and Nutrition

Margaret McLaren, RD

Publisher: Robert H. Garrison, Jr., MA, RPh

Editor In Chief: Elizabeth Somer, MA, RD

Managing Editor: Lisa M. Moye

Editorial Director: Janet L. Haley

Art Director: Scott Mayeda

Production Directors: Jeff Elkind, Irene Villa, Becky Moyer

Copy Editors: Norma Trost Foor, Jean Forsythe, Mary Houser, Stephen C. Schneider, R. H. Garrison, Sr.

Cover Design: Stefanko & Hetz, Jeff Elkind

Photography: Bob and Irene Nishihira, Carlsbad, CA

Illustration: Jennifer Hewitson, Julian Naranjo, Walter Stuart

Copyright © 1986 by Health Media of America, Inc.

For information regarding volume purchase discounts contact:
Health Media of America, Inc.
11300 Sorrento Valley Road, Suite 250
San Diego, CA 92121

Printed in the United States of America.

ISBN 0-937325-07-4

Contents

Introduction

Introduction

CONGRATULATIONS! You have taken the first step in a successful weight loss program by picking up this book. It shows you are interested in both weight control and good nutrition. This is probably not the first time you have tried to lose weight. Many people choose temporary ''weight loss regimes'' and have varying degrees of success. Many people have lost weight only to gain it again, sometimes gaining even more than was lost. Excess weight can be lost and a healthy weight can be maintained if a realistic and individualized program of nutrition and exercise is established for life.

In WEIGHT LOSS AND NUTRITION, you will learn about the scientific basis for obesity, the current treatment methods, and how to plan a weight control program. The health risks associated with overweight also are discussed. This book does not come with a money back guarantee that you will lose weight. There are no simple answers to weight loss, but, this book provides the tools necessary to make a weight loss program work for you.

1
Why Do People Gain Weight?

Obesity is an excess of body fat in relation to muscle and other lean tissues. Obesity reflects a long-term imbalance in the amount of calories consumed in the diet and the amount of calories used in physical activity and maintenance of body processes. Development of obesity, however, is more complicated than just calories in versus calories out. Obesity is a complex issue and is caused by a combination of physiological, psychological, and sociological factors that begin in childhood and are reinforced throughout life.

The types of obesity can be divided into two categories: obesity caused by an excess consumption of calories and obesity caused by an internal imbalance. As evidence accumulates it might be accepted that most cases of obesity are a result of internal imbalances and that calorie consumption is secondary to these imbalances.[1] This does not mean that obesity is incurable. It does mean that an overweight person who eats little food and struggles to lose weight should not feel guilty or ashamed for ''lack of will power.'' Regardless of the origin of obesity, there are guidelines to lose excess weight and maintain weight loss.

Several theories provide information on how and why some people are more prone to overweight than

1

other people. These theories include genetics, environmental influences, hormonal and glandular factors, the brown fat theory, the enzyme theory, the set point theory, the fat cell theory, and carbohydrate imbalances.

The Genetics Theory

A tendency to gain excess weight might be inherited. Children of obese parents have a greater likelihood of becoming overweight then do children of normal weight parents.[2] A child of normal weight parents has approximately a 10% chance of becoming overweight as an adult. For the child with one overweight parent, the chance is about 40%, and for the child with two overweight parents the likelihood of obesity increases to 80%. Studies on identical twins and non-identical twins show that weight gain might be a result of genetic factors.[3] *(Graph 1, Page 3)*

Animals are used as test-models when researchers try to understand certain conditions in humans. Some animals that have a high risk for obesity also have larger and greater quantities of fat cells than leaner animals. This type of condition could occur in some overweight people and could be a result of changes in the genetic code that programs the growth and development of fat cells.[4] The genetically altered fat tissue might cause more fat to be stored in the fat cell rather than burned for energy.

These abnormally large fat cells also are resistant to insulin. Insulin is a hormone produced by the pancreas that regulates the cells' use of sugar (glucose). Glucose is the end product of food digestion and the source of energy used by the body. Because the cells do not respond to insulin, the pancreas is given the

2

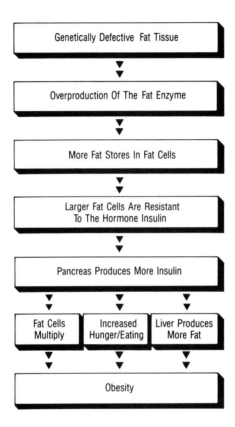

Graph 1. Model For Genetic Obesity

signal to produce more insulin. A high insulin production:

- Stimulates hunger and eating;
- Stimulates the liver to produce more fat;
- Causes the fat cells to multiply.

These genetic influences on weight gain are more likely to occur in the person who is overweight from childhood.[3]

The Environment Theory

The most popular theory of obesity states that overweight is a result of the environment.[5-9] For example, a person might consume more calories than he or she requires to maintain weight because of one or more of the following:

- The behavior was learned from the parents;
- A person responds to feelings such as stress and boredom by eating;
- A person over-reacts to outside cues such as television commercials;
- A person receives an inadequate amount of exercise;
- A person lacks discipline or "will power"; or
- A person is susceptible to pressure from friends and relatives to overindulge.

The environment theory states that behaviors are learned and that eating patterns that promote weight gain are reinforced by environmental cues and pressures. Behaviors also can be "unlearned" or replaced by new behaviors that promote weight loss and weight maintenance. The Behavior Modification approach to weight control is based on this theory.

The Fat Cell Theory

The number of fat cells in the body might result from overeating early in life rather than genetics.[10,11] Fat tissue can expand in two ways: an increase in the number of fat cells or an increase in the size of fat cells.

During infancy, childhood, adolescence, and pregnancy, growth is rapid and both the number and size of fat cells increase. Once fat cells are formed they are not destroyed, but their size can increase or decrease during the adult years.

When excess calories are consumed they are stored in fat tissue and the individual fat cells become larger. When weight is lost, the fat cells "shrink" to normal size. If overeating persists during a growth period the fat cells increase in size and number *(Graph 2)*.

Weight loss can reduce the size of the fat cell but not the number of cells. The overfed child or adolescent has more fat cells and a greater tendency for obesity later in life.[12]

The Fat Cell theory also might explain why some women have difficulty losing weight after pregnancy.

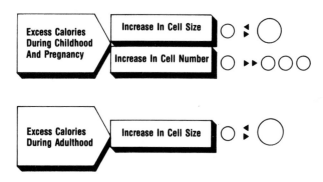

Graph 2. The Fat Cell Theory

The Fat Cell Theory states that overeating during critical growth periods results in an increase in the number and size of fat cells. The size can be reduced with diet and exercise, but the number of fat cells cannot be changed.

The "Gland/Hormone Problem" Theory

Obesity usually is not caused by "a gland problem." Less than 3% of all cases of overweight can be attributed to the glands, such as "underactive thyroid gland."[2] However, there are several glands that might be related to obesity, including the hypothalamus gland.

The Hypothalamus: The hypothalamus is a gland located in the base of the brain. The hypothalamus can regulate body temperature, emotional state, many body organ functions, and appetite.

The Appetite Center is located in the hypothalamus gland.[13] This center controls how much food a person eats and when it is eaten. The Center receives messages of hunger from the stomach that signal a person to eat. It sends messages to other parts of the brain that signal a person to stop eating when full. When one portion of the Appetite Center is damaged a person is more likely to overeat. When another portion of the Appetite Center is damaged a person is not hungry and is likely to lose weight to the point of self-starvation.[3] *(Figure 1, Page 7)*

Insulin: Insulin is a hormone secreted by the pancreas that regulates blood sugar levels. Food intake increases when people are injected with insulin.[14] Since insulin lowers the blood sugar level it might increase the desire to eat.

Estrogen: Estrogen is another hormone that might influence weight gain by its effect on food intake. Estrogen is the female hormone that regulates ovulation. When estrogen is given to animals, they eat less. When estrogen levels are low, eating resumes and the animal gains body fat.[14] Estrogen levels fluctuate during the menstrual cycle, but whether

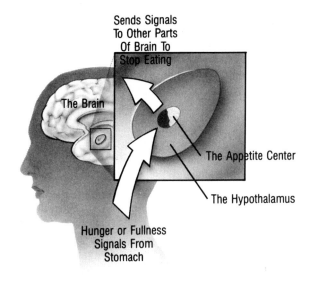

Sends Signals
To Other Parts
Of Brain To
Stop Eating

The Brain

The Appetite Center

The Hypothalamus

Hunger or Fullness
Signals From
Stomach

Figure 1. The Appetite Center is located in the hypothalamus gland in the brain. This center controls appetite.

changes in eating patterns reflect these fluctuations is unknown.

Cholescystokinin (CCK): CCK is a hormone secreted by the upper small intestine in response to food. This hormone might send signals to the brain that food intake is adequate. When animals are given this hormone, food intake stops.[15]

Other hormones involved in the control of eating and weight maintenance include growth hormone from the pituitary gland in the brain and thyroxin from the thyroid gland. If there is an upset in the production or use of either of these hormones, overweight could result.[16-18]

The Brown Fat Theory

Body weight is a reflection of calories in balanced by calories out. However, some people overeat and gain weight, while others overeat and do not gain weight. This observation implies that in some people energy or calories are "lost" rather than stored as fat.

Most calories from the diet are used to maintain body functions such as hair growth, heartbeat, breathing, and digestion. Another portion of the daily calorie intake is used to fuel physical activity such as walking, shopping, or cooking. Some calories are used to produce heat (thermogenesis), a process that includes a specific type of fat called brown adipose tissue (BAT) or brown fat.

There are different types of body fat. Most fat tissues (white fat) store fat and release it as needed for energy. About 1% of body fat is brown fat. Brown fat does not release fats into the blood stream for energy use by other tissues. Brown fat tissues burn fat to produce heat that maintains body temperature and keeps a person warm. This energy is "wasted" because the fat and its calories are not stored but are continually used for heat production. Some overweight people might have less brown fat, or the brown fat they have is not as active.[19]

The loss of energy or heat after eating is called "diet-induced thermogenesis." Animals with a tendency for obesity have defective brown fat. They do not convert food into body heat, but store it as fat. They become obese in spite of a normal food intake.[20]

Alterations in brown fat might contribute to obesity in some people. Differences between obese and non-obese people in diet-induced thermogenesis is most pronounced when the diet is high in fat.[21] Normal weight people, compared to overweight people,

8

produce more heat as a result of eating the same amount of calories. In addition, when the normal weight person overeats, the heat produced during digestion, absorption, and utilization of food is increased to compensate for the overload. This is not observed in the overweight individual.[12,19,22-25]

The brown fat or diet-induced thermogenic response to eating might explain why some people can overeat and not gain weight, while others cannot. In addition, the amount of heat lost is related to the total surface area of the body. A tall, lean person has more surface area in body mass and loses more heat than a short, heavy person. *(Figure 2, Page 10)*

The Enzyme Theory

Enzymes are protein-like substances in the body that regulate all chemical reactions. For example, enzymes dissolve food during digestion, facilitate the formation of proteins and all substances in the cells, and convert carbohydrates to energy. One theory of weight gain states that some people might have more enzymes that deposit fat into fat tissue and "lock" it into the tissue. These people might be more prone to obesity than leaner people who have more enzymes that remove fat from fat tissue and burn it for energy.

Obese people might use blood sugar for energy, rather than a mixture of sugar and fat. When sugar stores are used, the obese person experiences low blood sugar and is hungry more often than the leaner person who burns a combination of fat and sugar.[26] Exercise might alter these enzyme levels in obese people to resemble the enzyme concentrations of lean people.[27]

One theory shows that aerobic exercise, such as walking, jogging, swimming, or bicycling, might alter

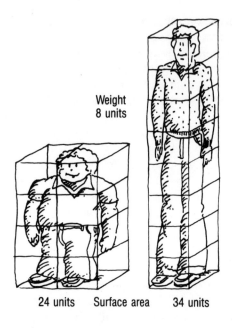

Weight
8 units

24 units   Surface area   34 units

Figure 2. The amount of heat lost is related to the total surface area of the body. A tall, lean person has a greater surface area than a short, heavy person and will lose more heat.

the enzymes of an obese person; weight is lost and maintained because extra calories are burned and the enzymes are changed to encourage weight maintenance.[27]

The Set Point Theory

The Set Point Theory states that all living organisms have a predetermined fat reserve that will be defended no matter what the challenge. For example, animals that are starved, or overfed to the point of obesity, return to their previous fat storage level and "normal weight" when allowed to regulate their own diets.[10]

This set point for body fat might be found in humans and would account for the ability of some people to lose weight, but not maintain the weight loss. The body loses weight in the "starvation" or dieting period and gains back the fat stores in an effort to return to what the body considers "normal."

Some people might have an abnormally high set point that interferes with permanent weight loss. Whereas the restriction of calories apparently cannot overcome a high set point, physical activity, especially aerobic exercise, might lower a person's set point and provide the means for permanent weight loss.[28]

Carbohydrate Balance Theories

Carbohydrates have been promoted as high calorie foods that encourage weight gain.[29-30] This is not true for all carbohydrates. The dietary recommendations for Americans to reduce the incidence of obesity, cardiovascular disease, diabetes, hypertension, and cancer suggest an increase in the consumption of complex carbohydrates.[31]

Carbohydrate foods are divided into two categories: simple carbohydrates or sugars, and complex carbohydrates or starch. Foods high in simple carbohydrates are candy, syrups, cookies, pie, and sweets. Complex carbohydrate foods are rice, pasta, whole and refined grain products, dried beans and peas, and starchy vegetables. The complex carbohydrates, especially the unrefined selections, provide protein, fiber, vitamins, and minerals as well as starch. Carbohydrates provide a readily available source of energy to the body.

The carbohydrate theory of weight control states that the Appetite Center *(Figure 1, Page 7)* in the hypothalamus and specialized cells in the liver are sensitive to the level of glucose in the blood.[3,10] A diet high in sugar (simple carbohydrate) might upset appetite regulation. When blood sugar levels are elevated, the Appetite Center and specialized liver cells signal the brain that the person is full and the person stops eating. When levels are low, messages are sent to the brain that it is time to eat.[3,10]

This theory might explain why some people overeat. Appetite and hunger might be a result of the carbohydrate content of the diet. After food is eaten, the hormone insulin is released to help transport the blood sugar glucose into the cells for nourishment. The amount of insulin released is related to the amount of carbohydrate consumed; the more carbohydrate, the greater the amount of insulin released. When blood sugar is adequate, a person feels satisfied. When blood sugar drops, a person feels hungry.

Hunger increases as the insulin transports the sugar out of the blood and into the cells. This process is exaggerated when the dietary carbohydrate is sugar. A person might feel weak, anxious, or uneasy because of low blood sugar. Soon after ingestion of a sugary food such as a candy bar, a person might feel better. The feelings of hunger and weakness return, however, within an hour or two when the simple sugar has been quickly digested, absorbed, and removed from the blood by insulin.[32]

Complex carbohydrates or starch are digested and absorbed slowly. They do not cause the rapid rise in blood sugar that is seen with sugar and so do not trigger excess insulin secretion and the drop in blood sugar.

Some people might be "carbohydrate cravers" because of the calming effect or drowsiness these people experience after eating a meal high in carbohydrates.[33] This relaxation might be a result of the effects of insulin or insulin and serotonin.

Serotonin is a hormone-like compound produced in the brain from the amino acid tryptophan. Serotonin regulates mood, sleep, pain, and other behaviors. Tryptophan must cross the lining of the intestine and then travel to the brain before it is available for conversion to serotonin.

Tryptophan competes with other amino acids for entry into the brain. In the presence of a high protein meal only moderate amounts of this amino acid enter the brain. A high carbohydrate/low protein meal helps remove amino acids that compete with tryptophan for entry into the brain; more tryptophan enters the brain and the synthesis of serotonin in the brain increases.[34] This might improve sleep and cause the drowsiness reported by some people after a carbohydrate meal.

If a person is a carbohydrate craver, he or she might want to include enough complex carbohydrate in the diet to maintain a level of comfort.[33]

Summary

One in every three people is overweight.[3] The possible causes of obesity are diverse and complex and vary from one person to another. It is certain, however, that weight gain is more than just a balance of calories in from food versus calories out as activity. Many people consume excess calories; not all of them are overweight. Heredity, individual differences in metabolism, and variations in how people use the calories they consume are important in weight control.

Regardless of the internal or external obstacles, most people can lose weight and maintain the weight loss. The successful approach to weight control must be an individualized program based on realistic weight loss goals. It might be unrealistic for a person who is very heavy to attain and maintain a very thin figure, but a desirable weight loss and weight maintenace that will last for life can be obtained with healthy eating habits and exercise.

2
Losing Weight: The Options

How Important Is The Diet?

Diet is what a person eats and everyone is constantly on a diet. Some diets are better than others because they taste good and promote good health. The word diet, however, is often mistaken to mean a temporary deviation from a person's normal food intake in an attempt to lose weight. Once the weight is lost, the "diet" is abandoned and a person returns to his or her normal food intake. The word diet has developed a bad name because of this association with quick, and often restrictive, weight loss programs.

Quick Weight Loss Diets: Why They Do Not Work

Hundreds of different techniques have been proposed as the "sure way" for people to lose weight. In many cases, a quick weight loss diet promotes an outdated weight loss theory under a new name.[35]

The success of the business of quick weight loss and the constant evolution of new fad diets occurs because the success rate for these diet plans is low; 95% of people who lose weight on a fad diet gain the weight back within the first year.[36] Because the long-term effects of quick weight loss diets are poor, a new diet is frequently promoted that promises an easy and painless way to lose weight.

15

Quick weight loss diets are popular for several reasons:

- People want to believe the diet will work. Losing and maintaining weight is not easy. People become discouraged by the failure of other more traditional methods of weight loss and are willing to try anything.
- It is human nature to look for the easy way out of a problem, to want something for nothing, and "to avoid the effort, frustration, and risk of failure that is essential to success."[37,38] *(Table 1, Page 17)*

The following are a few fad diet plans that perpetuate the myth of an easy answer to weight loss.

Fasting and Low-Calorie Diets: When the body is deprived of adequate calories it uses its own stores of fat and protein to provide the energy to maintain body functions. It will not exclusively use fat tissue. After less than twenty-four hours on a fast, the body begins to use muscle stores as a source of energy.[39] This causes a loss of muscle and other lean tissues and organs.

The hazards of fasting or very low-calorie diets include ketosis, dehydration, increased uric acid blood levels, nausea, dizziness, fatigue, and possible heart, kidney, or liver failure. A diet of less than 1,200 to 1,500 calories does not provide adequate amounts of essential nutrients and does not promote long-term habit change or weight loss.[36] A fasting or low-calorie diet should only be followed under the supervision of a physician.

Modified Fasting Diets: Nutrient supplemented liquids, powders, and protein beverages are a modifi-

Table 1   Myths About Weight Loss

In addition to the fad diets, a person must be alert to the fallacies that surround weight reduction. The American Dietetic Association has collected data on food misinformation. These were commonly-held fallacies related to weight control:

1. Obesity is due entirely to heredity.

2. In the experience of some people, all foods turn to fat.

3. Meal skipping is a good way to lose weight.

4. You can eat all you want and still lose weight if you take "reducing pills."

5. Special low calorie bread should be used in reducing diets.

6. Toast has fewer calories than bread.

7. One must not drink water when trying to lose weight.

8. Candy enriched with vitamins may be eaten when a person is reducing.

9. Washing rice after cooking reduces calories.

10. Sugar is not as fattening as starch.

11. High protein foods and fruits have no calories.

12. Gelatin dessert is nonfattening.

13. Milk should not be included in a weight reduction diet.

14. Meat burns its own calories.

15. Margarine contains fewer calories than butter.

16. For reducing, eat high protein foods for a week; then eat anything you want for a week.

17. Grapefruit will reduce a person's weight.

Source: Food Facts Talk Back. Chicago, The American Dietetic Association, 1957.

cation of fasting. The adverse effects of these diets vary according to each approach, but can include the same problems as are seen in fasting and low-calorie diets. Liquid protein supplemented fasts have been successful with medical supervision. Without this supervision there is a risk of sudden death from changes in body metabolism.[36,40]

High Protein/Low Carbohydrate Diet: People might lose weight quickly on this diet, but the weight loss is not maintained. If more than four pounds are lost in one week, the weight loss is probably loss of water and protein (muscle) with a minor amount of fat loss. The weight loss is a result of the reduced calorie intake, not the type of foods consumed or their proposed effects on fat metabolism. In addition, high protein/low carbohydrate diets raise blood levels of cholesterol and other fats and increase a person's risk for developing cardiovascular disease. High protein-low carbohydrate diets are unsafe because of the added stress they place on the kidneys to excrete the waste products of excessive protein intake.[36,41]

Diets That Alter Metabolism: Several quick weight loss diets promote one food or a combination of foods to increase metabolism. A person supposedly will use more calories without increasing physical activity. For example, one diet advises that grapefruit be consumed before each meal because grapefruit "burns fat." There is no evidence that this is true. The fallacy of this theory is reflected in the poor success rate of this type of diet.[36]

Enzyme diets claim that a combination of foods will change the body's metabolism and "melt" fat. These foods might be something as simple as eggs or fruits, or something as complex as lecithin, vitamin B_6, kelp, and vinegar. If a person loses weight on

18

these diets it is because of a reduction in calorie intake, not because of any effect of the foods.

Cellulite Diets: Cellulite diets are based on the theory that there are different kinds of fat. Cellulite is labeled as the type of fat that causes the thighs and buttocks to ripple or bulge. Cellulite theorists claim cellulite contains toxic wastes and cellular breakdown products. There is no such fat as cellulite. Fat tissue is the same no matter where it is located in the body. The rippling is caused by strands of connective tissue that tie the fat cells to underlying layers of tissue below the skin. When fat cells increase in size, the compartments of fat bulge between the strands and cause the appearance of rippling.

Summary: There is no special food, no magic combination of foods, and no formula that will increase weight loss. Grapefruit does not ''burn'' calories, protein foods do not cause permanent weight loss any faster than carbohydrate foods, and the order in which foods are ingested does not affect weight. What does affect the maintenance of normal weight is an individualized low-calorie, nutritious diet combined with regular exercise. The diet and exercise plan is only successful if the weight is lost and the weight loss is maintained.

The Dietary Recommendations Of National Nutrition Groups

Most Americans should increase consumption of high fiber foods such as fresh fruits and vegetables and whole grain breads and cereals, and reduce consumption of fatty meats, fatty dairy foods, and foods high in salt.[31,42-44] *(Graph 3, Page 20)*

The average diet provides 66% of its calories from foods high in fat and sugar and low in vitamins and

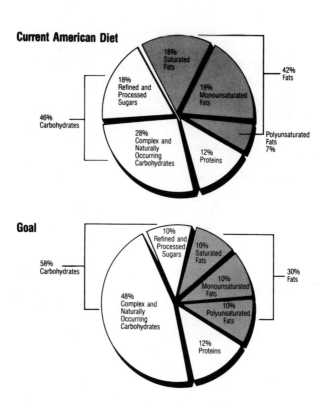

Current American Diet

16% Saturated Fats

19% Monounsaturated Fats

42% Fats

Polyunsaturated Fats 7%

12% Proteins

18% Refined and Processed Sugars

46% Carbohydrates

28% Complex and Naturally Occurring Carbohydrates

Goal

10% Refined and Processed Sugars

10% Saturated Fats

10% Monounsaturated Fats

10% Polyunsaturated Fats

30% Fats

58% Carbohydrates

48% Complex and Naturally Occurring Carbohydrates

12% Proteins

Graph 3. The U.S. Dietary Goals

minerals.[31] Favorite foods are coffee, margarine, doughnuts, soft drinks, eggs, and hamburgers.[45]

These food choices increase the fat, sugar, cholesterol, and salt content of the diet and might increase a person's chances of developing cardiovascular disease, cancer, diabetes, and hypertension.[31] Even the normal weight person who consumes this high-fat, low-fiber diet is at increased risk for these degenerative diseases.[31,44,46] The risk is increased when a person is overweight. Diet is very important for the prevention and treatment of these disorders for both the normal weight and the overweight person.

In addition to the fat, sugar, salt, cholesterol, and fiber content in the diet, major national nutrition surveys show that diets in the United States are not well-balanced in vitamins and minerals. Deficiencies of vitamin A, vitamin C, vitamin B_1, vitamin B_2, vitamin B_6, calcium, chromium, iron, and magnesium are prevalent.[47-52] If fatty foods are reduced and fiber foods are increased, the risk decreases for developing obesity, the degenerative diseases, and nutrient deficiencies.

The Dietary Fat Issue: Most dietary recommendations advocate a low-fat diet. The US Dietary Goals and the American Heart Association recommend that the current consumption of 42% of total calories as fat be reduced to less than 30%.[31,53] A reduction in total fat intake would reduce the risk for obesity. *(Figure 3, Page 22)*

Fat provides more than twice the calories of carbohydrates (starch and sugar) and protein and is a concentrated source of calories. When fat is reduced in the diet, calories are reduced. A baked potato supplies about 100 calories; sour cream and butter can double or triple the calorie content. Fried chicken contains more than twice the calories of baked chicken without the skin, although both are the same size.

The Fiber Issue: A high-fiber diet, comprised mainly of fresh fruits and vegetables, dried beans and peas, whole grain breads and cereals, and moderate amounts of foods from animal sources is linked to a reduced risk for cancer and other degenerative

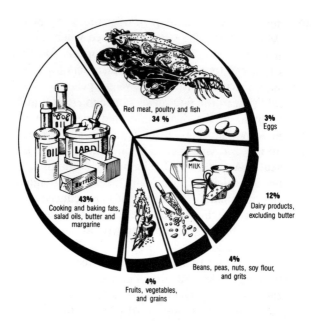

Figure 3. Sources of Fat In The American Diet

A reduction in dietary fat would reduce the risk of developing obesity, cardiovascular disease, cancer, diabetes and hypertension.

disorders.[31,42,43,54] In addition, fiber foods are low in fat and calories and high in vitamins and minerals. An individual can eat a greater quantity of fiber foods but consume fewer calories than if the diet includes many fatty foods. Fiber adds bulk to the diet, which helps satisfy hunger pangs without exceeding the days' calorie allotment.

The Sugar Issue: The average American eats almost 100 pounds of sugar each year. That is more than a quarter of a pound of sugar or over 400 calories each day. Much of this sugar is from soft drinks.[55]

Sugary foods are a poor substitute for more nutritious foods. Sugary foods either replace these foods in the diet, which might result in malnutrition, or are added to the normal food intake, which might encourage excess weight gain. *(Figure 4)*

The Good News: While some foods should be limited in the diet, a variety of other foods can be substituted in their place. Dietary recommendations for the prevention of disease, obesity, and nutrient deficiencies state that people should increase their consumption of fresh fruits and vegetables, whole grain breads and cereals, dried beans and peas and other fiberous foods, and consume moderate amounts of lean meat, chicken, fish, and low-fat dairy foods. These foods supply vitamins, minerals, fiber, and protein and a moderate amount of fat and calories.

Behavior Modification

Behavior modification is an approach to weight loss and maintenance that includes the behaviors related to eating, the selection of food, and discontinuation of "overeating." It establishes a plan for

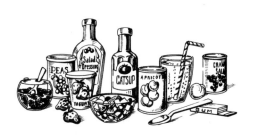

Figure 4.   Hidden Sugars In Foods

modifiying behaviors to lose weight and maintain normal weight.[56,57] The primary goal of behavior modification is establishing healthy eating habits; it does not focus on weight loss, although this is the desired result.

This psychological approach to weight control has three core characteristics.[8]

- The person makes an assessment of his or her eating and activity habits. The environmental cues that might influence these patterns are considered.
- Certain negative behaviors are targeted for change or elimination and a system of self-monitoring is developed.
- Instruction and guidance on the replacement of the old negative responses or behaviors with new positive responses or behaviors is emphasized.

A person is more likely to lose weight and maintain that weight loss when these principles are part of the diet program.[8,56,58,59]

The Role Of Exercise In Weight Loss

Weight loss programs that incorporate exercise with diet are more effective than diet alone.[60-67] Summarized below are the benefits of exercise and diet combined.

Increased Muscle Mass: Regular exercise builds muscle. It takes more calories to maintain muscle tissue than to maintain fat tissue. As muscle is developed, a person can consume the same or more food and lose weight because of both the calories burned during the exercise and the calories used between exercise sessions to maintain the muscle. A restricted calorie diet without exercise reduces muscle.

Increased Basal Metabolic Rate (BMR): BMR is the number of calories used to maintain basic functions. BMR accounts for about 60% of a person's allowable calorie intake. Anytime the BMR is raised, more calories are burned. A higher BMR means faster weight loss. BMR decreases when food intake is low. A calorie-restricted diet, without exercise, might not result in weight loss because of its suppressive effect on BMR. There is also the possibility that exercise can raise the BMR and keep it higher for hours later.

Reduced Fat Stores: Exercisers use fat stores instead of muscle stores as a source of energy.

Increased Energy Level: Exercise increases feelings of well-being. Diet alone often causes a feeling of mild depression. A person might restrict movement even further because the body is reacting to a "starvation" state.

Suppressed Appetite: Moderate exercise reduces appetite. Extreme exercise might increase appetite but only in proportion to the amount of energy used. Weight loss is still the result.[64]

Increases Overall Fitness And Stamina: This is especially true with regular aerobic activity. The heart pumps more efficiently.

Reduced Blood Pressure: Regular exercise lowers the heart rate and reduces blood pressure.[67]

Decreased Anxiety: Exercise might reduce tension and is a healthy alternative to overeating. Studies also show that dieting itself is a stressful situation.[64,68]

Increased Use Of Calories: Exercise increases the amount of calories burned each day. A person can lose weight with no change in calorie intake if exercise is included in the daily routine. *(Figure 5, Page 26)*

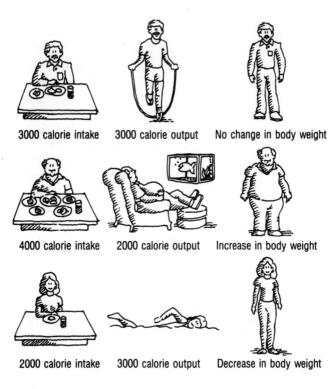

3000 calorie intake 3000 calorie output No change in body weight

4000 calorie intake 2000 calorie output Increase in body weight

2000 calorie intake 3000 calorie output Decrease in body weight

Figure 5. A person can lose weight without a drastic reduction in calories when exercise is included in the daily routine.

Normalized Blood Sugar: Obese people can have decreased sensitivity to the action of insulin. Although the pancreas produces enough insulin, the cell's do not respond to the insulin by absorbing the blood sugar so that it can be converted to energy. Regular exercise can improve insulin sensitivity and help maintain normal blood sugar levels.[69]

Lowered Set Point: The set point might be lowered with regular exercise.[66] Exercise might be an effective way to pass plateaus in weight loss and maintain weight loss.

Summary

The goal of a weight program is not only weight loss. Attainment and maintenance of desired weight is most important. Overweight is a complex behavioral and physiological issue; there is no single cause for its development and no one solution for its cure. However, there are two components necessary for any weight loss and weight maintenance plan: diet and exercise.

Permanent weight loss, or more precisely fat loss, can only occur with a combination of diet and exercise. Extreme calorie restriction alone places a person at risk for developing nutrient deficiencies. Exercise will increase calorie loss during and between exercise sessions and allow a person to eat more food and nutrients than if only diet is used to lose weight.

3
Planning The Weight Control Program

The Assessment

A personal health record needs to be developed for an individual planning a weight loss program.

Step 1: On a sheet of paper, write the reasons why you want to lose weight. Be honest. This step is important and might take several days to complete. Making a lifestyle change such as weight loss requires commitment. That commitment is based on a clear understanding of why the change is important to you.

Step 2: Use Table 2 *(Page 29)* to record body measurements. Be sure to take into consideration your correct frame size. *(Table 3, Page 30)* Check the Height and Weight Table *(Table 4, Page 40)* and include the weight that corresponds with your frame size in the record. Fill in the Goal Weight blank after reading the section on The Weight Loss Goal.

Step 3: Use the Habit Inventory Test *(Table 5, Page 41)* to assess food and eating behaviors. The Food Selection Analysis *(Table 6, Page 42)* can be used to assess attitudes toward certain kinds of food.

Evaluate your food selection and behavior by examining your answers on the Habit Inventory Test. There are no "bad" behaviors; however, some behaviors might interfere with weight loss and weight maintenance. The areas that promote poor eating habits should be targeted for improvement as you design your plan for reaching your weight loss goal.

Table 2   Body Measurements

Measurement	Start Date	1 Month	2 Months	3 Months	4 Months
Height					
Weight					
Frame Size					
Chest					
Waist					
Hip					
Right Thigh					
Left Thigh					

Ideal Weight Range _____ (See Table 4)

Goal Weight Range _____

Goal Date _____

Step 4: The Food Diary *(Table 7, Page 43)* is important in a weight loss program. Information in the Food Diary should be accurate and complete. Make several copies of this sheet and record food and beverage intake for seven days. Estimate portion sizes. Record mood while eating. Do not leave any blanks. During the first week consume your regular diet. Do not try to restrict food intake. You are focusing on usual eating habits.[70]

Table 3   Body Frame Size

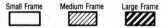

Small Frame Medium Frame Large Frame

Use height without shoes and inches for wrist size to determine frame size from this chart.

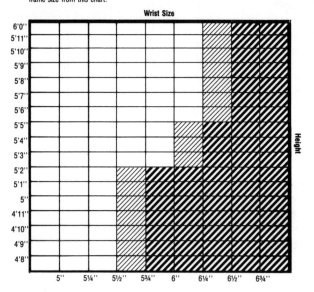

Wrist Size

Step 5: Use Table 8 *(Page 44)* to determine the daily calorie allotment necessary to maintain your current weight. Fill out the portion on the chart that applies to your goal weight after reading the section entitled The Weight Loss Goal.

The initial assessment will provide the reasons for losing weight and current information on your body measurements, eating habits and attitudes, and calorie intake. It is the foundation for making changes.

The Weight Loss Goal

A realistic goal must be determined before a weight loss program is started. Numerous factors should be considered in determining that goal including family history of weight gain, current lifestyle habits, resources available to begin and continue a weight control program, age, and medical history. Goals should be:

- Realistic
- Controllable
- Specific And Easily Measured
- Flexible
- Progressively More Challenging

Be Realistic: A comparison of your present weight with the Height-Weight Table is not the measure of ideal body weight. The weight at which you feel most comfortable might be closer to your ideal body weight.[71] *(Figure 6, Page 32)*

Be realistic and thorough in establishing a goal and keep an image in your mind of the person you would like to be in terms of weight and health.

Stay In Control: Set a goal that you can control. You can establish an exercise program, but a goal that requires you to exercise with your spouse is not under your control. If your spouse does not want to exercise every day, you fail. A goal should depend only on you.

Be Specific: A clear image of the "ideal" you is important in identifying the goal. "I will lose 10 pounds in two months by a program that includes exercising three times a week for one-half hour each

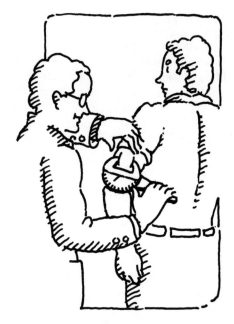

Figure 6. A skinfold test for percent body fat will assess current "fatness" and provide a baseline index for setting weight loss goals.

day" is specific. Weight may be only a minor or major part of that image.

Be Flexible: Part of a realistic goal is that it is flexible and provides for human error. If you exceed your calorie consumption or are unable to exercise on one day, do not give up the program. Start again the next day.

Be Progressive: Goals should be progressive. For example, if you want to lose seventy-five pounds, set small goals of five to ten pound increments. Small successes encourage and motivate a person to continue. Unrealistic goals can be discouraging.

The Weight Loss Plan

Fill in the goal Weight on Table 2 *(Page 29)* and complete the calculations for determining the calorie allotment for weight reduction and weight maintenance in Table 8 *(Page 44)*.

To determine the goal date for completion of weight loss, consider that no more than two pounds should be lost each week. A gradual weight reduction is healthier and more likely to be maintained than a quick weight loss.

After completing the seven day Food Diary, examine it for behavior patterns. Are you overeating when you are tired? Are you eating too fast? What are your unique behaviors? Take a colored pen and circle the behaviors that interfere with goal weight. Now make a list of the behaviors you want to change. Consider the information you identified in the Habit Inventory Test and Food Selection Analysis. Number the behaviors that need to be changed in order of importance to you.

Choose the top two or three behaviors that interfere with achieving your goal weight. For each of these behaviors list one or two new behaviors that would help you lose weight. For example, if you have identified that you overeat when food is served at the table, a new behavior would be to serve meals from the counter or stove and not to return for second helpings.

Set a time limit for the new behavior that is realistic and practical. If a behavior will be easy to change, the time limit might be one week. A difficult behavior change might take months.

Reward yourself when you have successfully incorporated a new behavior into your lifestyle. Do not use food as a reward. Instead, take a walk in the country, go to a movie, buy yourself a present, or take the day off. Continue to repeat the new behavior until it feels comfortable and is automatic, then identify another behavior to change.

If you do not succeed, re-evaluate your goal. Was it unrealistic? What interfered with success? Begin again. You can do it! *Table 9, Page 45)*

Thinking, Attitudes, And Wants: Barriers To Success

Thoughts: Your thinking will influence whether a weight loss program is successful. The key to success is personal responsibililty; you control your actions and choices. Thoughts of "I can't," "I should," or "I have to" will undermine the best weight loss plan. The foundation of all success is the belief that you can and that you will. Most important is the attitude that you choose to make these changes. If the thought "I can't get through the morning without my sweet roll" pops into your mind, replace it with "I can get through the morning and I choose to do so."

The "I don't care's" or "just this once's" are typical thoughts when faced with a tempting old behavior. You do care and can choose to stick with the new behavior rather than becoming a victim of temptation.

Attitudes: The Food Selection Analysis *(Table 6, Page 42)* is an attitude indicator. Are most of your favorite foods of the high-fat, high-sugar, or high-sodium type? What food do you use when you need comforting? How many of the foods you listed were really nutritious? Was the food you listed as healthy for you one that you eat and enjoy frequently? Do you find nutritious foods boring and the calorie-laden foods exciting?

It is common for people to reward themselves with non-nutritious food. Although there are no "bad" eating habits, there might be habits that are not useful for weight control.[40]

The identification of attitudes that encourage weight gain is useful for planning a strategy for change. A change in attitude toward eating might help overcome these habits. For example, if sugary or fatty foods are used as a reward for a hard day ("I deserve it") perhaps a change in attitude that supports the concept that you deserve the best, and only the most nutritious foods fit that description, would encourage low-calorie, nutritious food choices. You can still have an occasional sweet food, but to include them daily in the diet undermines your long-term goal.

Wants: Ignore your wants. You might not always want to stick with the program. That is expected, but it does not matter. Wanting or not wanting is irrelevant. The long-term goal is more important than your wants today. Choosing to stick with the program every day was part of the initial promise to yourself.[72]

The Diet

There are certain characteristics that make a weight reduction diet successful and practical. The diet should:

- offer a wide variety of foods, including fresh fruits and vegetables; whole grain breads and cereals; low-fat or nonfat dairy foods; and lean meat, chicken, fish, or dried beans and peas;
- be nutritionally balanced and provide a minimum of 1,200 calories, unless supervised by a physician;
- be based on personal food preferences;
- promote long-term habit change;
- include regular meals, at least three to six meals a day;
- include snacks;
- follow the Dietary Guidelines *(Page 20)*;
- be affordable and easy to follow;
- result in weight loss of about one to two pounds each week.

Is A Structured Diet Plan Best For You?

Some people need a structured diet plan to assure successful weight loss. Other people need general guidelines. Regardless of the diet you choose, record food intake in the Food Diary for the first month. This recordkeeping reinforces the commitment to lose weight and helps you monitor food intake, food behaviors, and food attitudes.

Calories are the main concern in any weight loss diet. Calories are contained in all foods. There are four dietary components that contain calories: protein, carbohydrate, alcohol, and fat.

- Protein supplies four calories/gram.
- Carbohydrates supply four calories/gram.
- Alcohol supplies seven calories/gram.
- Fat supplies nine calories/gram.

Weight is gained when excess calories, from any one or all of these dietary sources, are consumed;

however, a reduction in fat and fatty foods has the greatest effect on reducing calories in the diet.

Table 10 *(Page 46)* is an example of a low-fat, high-fiber, high-carbohydrate diet based on the Dietary Guidelines. Fat constitutes 30% of the total calories, carbohydrate (starch) constitutes 50% to 60% of total calories, and protein constitutes 10% to 15% of total calories. Portions should be weighed or measured until you can accurately estimate the size.

Foods should be baked, steamed, broiled, boiled, or poached rather than fried or sauteed. *(Table 11, Page 47)*

Food choices based on the guidelines listed in Table 10 *(Page 46)* should reflect personal preferences, time demands, and eating habits. They can be eaten in three "square meals" or divided into several small meals throughout the day.

Is An Unstructured Diet Plan Best For You?

The following guidelines can be used if counting calories and portion sizes does not work for you.

- Reduce or eliminate alcohol. Alcohol contains calories, but few nutrients. A person on a low-calorie diet cannot afford to waste calories on nutrient-poor foods. Wine can be used to flavor foods in cooking, since the alcohol (and its calories) are lost when foods are heated.
- Reduce consumption of fats and fatty foods. *(Figure 7, Page 38)*
- Eliminate or reduce sugars and sugary foods. *(Figure 4, Page 23)*
- Monitor portions.

37

- Two-thirds of the diet should include fresh fruits and vegetables, dried beans and peas, and whole grain breads and cereals. The other one-third of the diet should come from two servings a day each of nonfat or low-fat dairy foods and lean meat, chicken, or fish. Limit serving sizes to eight ounces of low-fat or nonfat milk, 1½ ounce low-fat cheese, and 2 to 3 ounces of meat, chicken, or fish.
- Bake, steam, broil, boil, or poach. Do not fry or saute. Eliminate or reduce intake of sauces, gravies, and "creamed" foods.

Vitamin-Mineral Supplementation

When the diet is less than 2,000 calories it is likely to be low in some vitamins and minerals.[50,51,52,73] A multiple vitamin-mineral supplement might be necessary to guarantee adequate nutrient intake.[74] Guidelines for choosing a supplement include:

- Choose a multiple vitamin-mineral supplement that contains the following nutrients:

The vitamins: vitamin A, vitamin E, vitamin D, vitamin B_1, vitamin B_2, niacin, vitamin B_6, folic acid,

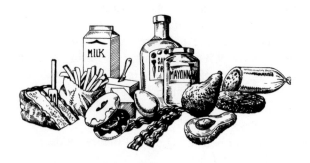

Figure 7. Foods High In Fat

38

vitamin B$_{12}$, pantothenic acid, biotin, and vitamin C.

The minerals: calcium, chromium, copper, iron, magnesium, manganese, molybdenum, selenium, and zinc. A separate supplement of calcium or magnesium might be required since a multiple vitamin-mineral preparation might not provide these minerals in adequate amounts.

- Choose a supplement that provides between one and three times the USRDA for each vitamin and mineral.

The Exercise Program

Exercise is essential to the success of a weight loss and weight maintenance program. The best type of exercise is the one you like and are willing to do. Aerobic exercise is preferred over anaerobic exercise because aerobic exercise will use the fat from fat tissue as its energy source; anaerobic exercise uses sugar stored in the muscles for energy. Examples of aerobic and anaerobic exericse are:

Aerobic	Anaerobic
Walking	Tennis
Swimming	Downhill Skiing
Bicycling	Badminton
Cross Country Skiing	Sprinting
Running	Weight Lifting
Trampoline	Racketball

It is easier to maintain an exercise and diet program when it is reinforced by other people. Join an organized group for exercise. Start slowly and gradually increase the intensity, frequency, and duration of exercise. If exercise is overdone, soreness or injury can discourage its continuation. The same behavior modification techniques used for dietary control will work with exercise.

Table 4   Height And Weight Tables

	Men				Women		
Height	Small frame	Med. frame	Lg. frame	Height	Small frame	Med. frame	Lg. frame
5'2"	128-134	131-141	138-150	4'10"	102-111	109-121	118-131
5'3"	130-136	133-143	140-153	4'11"	103-113	111-123	120-134
5'4"	132-138	135-145	142-156	5'0"	104-115	113-126	122-137
5'5"	134-140	137-148	144-160	5'1"	106-118	115-129	125-140
5'6"	136-142	139-151	146-164	5'2"	108-121	118-132	128-143
5'7"	138-145	142-154	149-168	5'3"	111-124	121-135	131-147
5'8"	140-148	145-157	152-172	5'4"	114-127	124-138	134-151
5'9"	142-151	148-160	155-176	5'5"	117-130	127-141	137-155
5'10"	144-154	151-163	158-180	5'6"	120-133	130-144	140-159
5'11"	146-157	154-166	161-184	5'7"	123-136	133-147	143-163
6'0"	149-160	157-170	164-188	5'8"	126-139	136-150	146-167
6'1"	152-164	160-174	168-192	5'9"	129-142	139-153	149-170
6'2"	155-168	164-178	172-197	5'10"	132-145	142-156	152-173
6'3"	158-172	167-182	176-202	5'11"	135-148	145-159	155-176
6'4"	162-176	171-187	181-207	6'0"	138-151	148-162	158-179

Weight at ages 25-59 in shoes and 5 pounds of indoor clothing.

Weight at ages 29-59 in shoes and 3 pounds of indoor clothing.

Source: Metropolitan Life Insurance.

Table 5   Habit Inventory Test

Directions: Answer the following questions according to how often you performed the activity in the past two weeks. Check "seldom" if the answer is seldom to never, "sometimes" if the answer is more than twice, and "frequently" if the answer is more than five times. Be honest. Answer all questions.

	Seldom	Some-times	Frequently
1. I engage in other activities while eating.	___	___	___
2. I put the utensils down between mouthfuls.	___	___	___
3. I leave food on the plate.	___	___	___
4. I store food out of sight.	___	___	___
5. I shop when hungry.	___	___	___
6. I eat slowly and enjoy each bite.	___	___	___
7. I eat when I am upset, depressed, or bored.	___	___	___
8. I substitute activities and exercise for eating.	___	___	___
9. I preplan my meals and snacks.	___	___	___
10. I only eat until I am full.	___	___	___
11. I think about food when I am not hungry.	___	___	___
12. I skip meals.	___	___	___
13. I eat because others are eating.	___	___	___
14. I snack between meals or taste food while cooking.	___	___	___
15. I use smaller plates and serve moderate portions.	___	___	___

Questions 1, 5, 7, 11, 12, 13, and 14 might promote poor eating habits if a person is trying to lose weight and engages in these activities more than once or twice a week. The other questions (2, 3, 4, 6, 8, 9, 10, and 15) foster eating habits that help a person lose weight and these habits should be practiced on a regular basis.

41

Table 6   The Food Selection Analysis
List The Food That Matches That Behavior:

1. The food you eat when celebrating.

_____

_____

_____

2. The food you eat when you are sad.

_____

_____

_____

3. The food you eat when you are mad.

_____

_____

_____

4. The food you eat when you are sick.

_____

_____

_____

5. Your favorite cultural food.

_____

_____

_____

6. The food you eat when you arrive home from work.

_____

_____

_____

7. The food you know is nutritious.

_____

_____

_____

8. Your favorite food.

_____

_____

_____

Table 7   The Food Diary

Date _____   Day of Week _____

Food Item & Portion	Time Spent Eating	Degree of Hunger*	Activity While Eating	Where Eating	Eating With Whom	Mood While Eating

* **Degree Of Hunger**   1   Not Hungry   2   Somewhat Hungry   3   Very Hungry

43

Table 8   **Calculate Calorie Needs**

To estimate your calorie needs, choose the factor under the column that corresponds to your sex and current activity level.

Activity level	Male	Female
Sedentary	16	14
Moderately active	21	18
Very active	26	22

Multiply this factor times your current weight to estimate your current calorie needs. Then multiply your goal weight times your goal activity factor to obtain the calorie intake required to maintain your goal weight. Deduct 500 calories/day to obtain the calories required to reach goal weight, assuming exercise level during weight loss matches the goal activity factor.

a. Present weight _____ × **Activity Factor** _____ = Calorie intake to maintain current weight.

b. Goal weight _____ × **Goal Activity Factor** _____ = Calorie intake to maintain goal weight once it is achieved.

c. Minus 500 calories = _____ Calories/day required to reach goal weight.

Example:

Current: 150 pounds sedentary woman × 14 = 2,100 calories.

Goal: 135 pounds moderately active woman × 18 = 2,430 calories.

To reach goal: 2,430 − 500 = 1,930 calories/day.

This is only an estimate of calorie needs.

Table 9   Practicing New Behaviors

What is the behavior you want to change?	When do you practice this behavior?	What NEW BEHAVIOR can you practice instead?	How often did you practice this NEW BEHAVIOR in the past week?				
			Never	Hardly Ever	Some-Times	Most Of The Time	Always
Example: Eating too fast	Lunch time at work	Take at least 20 minutes to eat					

Table 10   Dietary Guidelines For Weight Loss

Food Group	Portion	Portions Daily	Calories/ Portion
Fruit	1/2 cup, 1 medium	3	40
Vegetable	1/2 cup cooked, 1 cup raw	3	25
Whole grain bread, cereal, rice or pasta	1 slice, 1 tortilla, 1/2 cup cooked cereal, 1/2 cup rice or pasta	5	70
Lean meat, chicken, fish, dried beans and peas	3 oz. meat, chicken or fish, or 1/2 cup dried beans/peas	2	130
Low-fat or nonfat milk or yogurt	8 oz milk or yogurt	2	90
Fats	1 tsp butter, margarine, oil, mayonnaise; 1/8 avocado; 1 tbsp. oil & vinegar dressing	2 to 3	45
Total calories			**1,120**

Percentage of calories from fat		31%
Percentage of calories from carbohydrates		49%
Percentage of calories from protein		20%

Table 11	**Reducing Fat In The Diet**

The following are suggestions for reducing your fat consumption:

1. Bake, broil, steam, or poach foods. Do not saute, fry, or use gravies or sauces in cooking.

2. Cook meats at low temperatures to enhance fat removal.

3. Skim fat from broth before making gravies or soup stock.

4. Do not bread or flour meats. The flour will absorb excess fat.

5. Use non-stick pans, rather than oil or butter.

6. Saute in defatted chicken stock, rather than in oil or butter.

7. Use nonfat milk rather than whole milk or cream in cooking.

8. Reduce the oil by one-half in recipes.

9. Use jam or marmalade on toast instead of butter.

4
Beating The Odds

Dealing With Sabotage

It is estimated that 30% of all dieters encounter sabotage from either family or close friends.[75] Spouses are guilty of double messages and encouraging deviation from the diet. Family members or friends encourage overeating at social gatherings and holidays. Saying no gracefully can be difficult; however it can be done. In the beginning of a weight loss program, you might:

- Avoid social gatherings that provide too much temptation.

- Bring a support person, such as a a friend or spouse, to help you monitor eating habits.

- Plan ahead. Decide what you will say or do before the social gathering.

- Have the dinner at your house and cook only "acceptable" foods.

- Learn to say "no, thank you."

- Choose social gatherings where people are either eating "acceptable" foods or are supportive of your new diet habits.

- Ask people to support your new diet habits by encouraging you to stick to your diet.

- Develop a personal list of survival skills to be used against social pressures.

Becoming A Food Snob

There might be times when you stray from the the new dietary pattern. Stop thinking of it as "ruining your diet" because you had gravy with dinner. There isn't anything you cannot have occasionally. All foods are on a diet plan as long as the frequency and portion size are monitored. Be selective when choosing to stray. If ice cream is a favorite food, have a one scoop serving once a week or once every two weeks.

Ask yourself if the pleasure from eating that food is worth the extra cost in exercise. If it is, than go ahead and enjoy it. Watch the portion size. If you develop an attitude of denial and feel like you cannot do or have what you want, you set yourself up for failure. The new eating habits must be flexible and practical.

Dining Out, Holidays, And Special Occasions

A party or social event can be a tempting opportunity to stray from a new eating habit. Techniques for reducing temptation include:

- Plan to increase exercise either before or immediately following the occasion.
- Eat fewer calories earlier in the day to allow for a greater intake during the party.
- Let the host or hostess know that you are on a certain meal plan. Offer to bring a dish that can be shared with friends and is still part of your plan.
- Pay more attention to the conversation and make it a goal to talk with everyone there rather than tasting all the hors d'oeavres.

- Call your local health department or Heart Association and ask about a local guide to restaurants that serve low calorie foods.
- Split a meal with another person. *(Table 12, Page 51)*

Staying Positive

Frustration, depression, or feeling sorry for yourself is normal in a weight loss program. Accept the possibility of an occasional bad moment, but wallow in it for no more than a few moments. Negative thoughts foster more negative thoughts. Be determined to switch off the blues within a reasonable period of time. Make a list of the positive changes made since the new program started. Reward yourself, with non-food rewards, for a job well done. To avoid unnecessary frustration, weigh yourself no more than twice a week. Body weight fluctuates between 1/2 and 2 pounds daily and frequent weighings can be deceiving.

The Plateau

If you hit a plateau in your weight loss, stay positive. Analyze your food intake and exercise and diet habits. If you have not kept the Food Diary, make a commitment to do it faithfully for the next seven days. Re-evaluate your long-term and short-term goals.

Plateaus are a normal part of a weight loss program although the reason for plateaus is poorly understood. If your food intake and exercise has not changed, maintain the weight loss program for two to three weeks before taking action. Often, after a few weeks, you will begin to lose weight again. If

Table 12	Dining Out

To enjoy an evening out without abandoning new eating habits, select foods from the following:

Appetizers: fresh fruit and vegetables, seafood cocktail.

Soups: consomme, barley, vegetable soups, fruit soups.

Salads: salad bars, all types of fresh vegetable or fruit salads. No dressing unless lemon, low-calorie, or vinegar.

Breads: whole grain breads, sourdough or enriched rolls, bagels, corn tortillas, rye crisp, and matzos.

Vegetables: baked potato with chives, all vegetables, except fried, battered, or sauteed.

Meat, Chicken, Fish: lean meat, fish, or skinned chicken. Avoid goose, duck, prime cuts, and fried, battered, gravied, or sauteed dishes. Baked, steamed, and broiled meats are preferable.

Desserts: gelatins, fruit ices, fresh fruit, or angel food cake.

Beverages: nonfat milk, fruit or vegetable juice, mineral water, tea, or black coffee.

Words To Avoid: refried, creamed, cream sauce, au gratin, in cheese sauce, au lait, a la mode, prime, pot pie, au fromage, hollandaise, or crispy.

there have been no changes in the diet and exercise and after three weeks the plateau remains, increase the frequency, intensity, or duration of exercise or cut back on the number of times you allow yourself to splurge on desserts, oils, or alcohol.

Summary

Control of your weight is a complicated process. Variables in cause, health risks, weight loss methods, and success make it difficult to recommend a single formula for everyone. An individualized program of low-fat, low-sugar, high-fiber foods and regular aerobic exercise is the best way to lose weight and keep it off for life.

5
The Health Risks Of Obesity

Life Expectancy

Poor health associated with overweight has been linked to a reduction in life expectancy. This relationship is much stronger for the severely overweight person, those 30% or more above normal weight, than for those who are moderately overweight.[76]

The maintenance of ideal body weight or a weight that is slightly under ideal weight might reduce a person's risk for developing several diseases.[76] There are a number of health conditions associated with obesity:

- Accidents
- Cancer
- Diabetes
- Infertility
- Gall Stones
- Gout
- Heart Disease
- High Blood Pressure
- Surgery
- Intestinal Disorders
- Joint Stress
- Poor Self-Image
- Pregnancy Problems
- Respiratory Disease
- Skin Problems
- Stroke
- Menstruation Problems

When a person gains weight, blood pressure increases, blood fats (triglycerides and cholesterol) increase, blood sugar and the hormone that regulates blood sugar (insulin) are elevated, a person is more prone to bone and joint diseases such as osteoarthritis, and cancers of the breast, ovaries, and endometrium (lining of the uterus) are more common.[35] Many of these condition are reversed with weight loss and maintenance. For example, some types of diabetes and hypertension are successfully treated with weight loss.[35] The prevention, treatment, or reversal of these degenerative diseases would improve the quality, and perhaps the length, of life. *(Figure 8)*

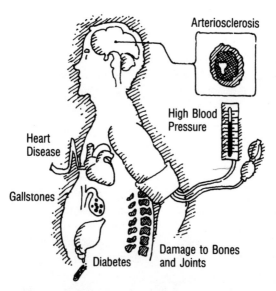

Figure 8. Consequences Of Obesity
When a person gains weight, blood pressure increases; blood fats increase (hear disease arteriosclerosis); blood sugar and insulin increase (diabetes); a person is prone to bone and joint disorders; and the likelihood increases for gallstone formation.

Cardiovascular Disease And High Blood Pressure

One out of every two people die from cardiovascular disease (CVD).[77] Cardiovascular disease includes atherosclerosis (hardening of the arteries), heart attacks, and strokes.

A primary risk factor for the development of atherosclerosis, heart disease, and stroke is elevated blood levels of cholesterol and high blood pressure (hypertension). The likelihood of developing cardiovascular disease (CVD) increases when the total cholesterol level is above 200 mg%.[44,53,76]

People who are overweight are more likely to have elevated blood fat levels than lean people.[78] If a person becomes obese during the middle years (ages 20 to 40 years old) the risk for developing CVD is higher than if weight gain occurs later in life.[76,79]

High blood pressure is also one of the major risk factors for CVD. As weight increases so does blood pressure.[76] A reduction of weight is one of the most effective means of lowering blood pressure.[68,80]

Diabetes

Over 10 million people have diabetes and the incidence of this disease is increasing.[81] Diabetes is the uncontrolled regulation of blood sugar, increased concentration of sugar in the blood, and increased excretion of sugar in the urine. Diabetics are more likely to develop CVD, kidney disease, eyesight problems, poor circulation that can lead to sores and gangrene, and increased susceptibility to infection.

Moderate obesity might increase by ten-fold the risk for developing diabetes. When overweight is more than 45% above normal, the risk increases to thirty-fold.[76] Often, weight loss alone returns blood sugar levels to normal.

Cancer

The American Cancer Society has established dietary guidelines for the prevention of cancer.[43] One of those guidelines is to maintain a normal body weight. The recommendation to avoid obesity is based on research that shows cancers of the uterus, gallbladder, kidney, prostate, cervix, stomach, colon, and breast are more frequent in obese than in nonobese people.[43,46,82,83]

People who maintain a normal body weight live longer and do not develop cancer as often as people who are overweight.[43] Low calorie diets also might reduce the risk of developing cancer, although this might be partially due to a reduction in dietary fat, a food component strongly linked to cancer.

The Impact Of Obesity On Emotional Stress

There have been very few studies that document the extent to which overweight people feel depression and anxiety specifically related to their weight.[84] The obese person often finds discrimination when applying for insurance, entering college, or applying for a job. Fashion trends also reflect the culture's emphasis on slimness.[85] These events might reinforce feelings of inadequacy and diminish self-esteem. This can result in a cycle of depression and low self-esteem that encourages eating for consolation, which results in additional weight gain, social or imagined disfavor, and a continued decline in self-esteem.[86]

Obese men and women do experience more muscle tension and anxiety over their body image than do normal weight people. A reduction in psychological stress and improvements in self- esteem are noted in obese people when they lose weight.[87]

The perception that one is overweight might produce more stress than the reality of obesity. One study showed that upper income young women who were not overweight according to the height-weight tables were more distressed about their weight than those who were clinically overweight.[79] In some cases, no difference is found between the mental health scores of overweight and normal weight people, but anxiety does increase in those people who are aggressively trying to lose weight.[88]

Many overweight people have experienced one or more of the following as a consequence of their weight:[5,62]

- Job Discrimination
- Social Isolation
- Public Ridicule
- Poor Self-Image
- Embarrassment
- Fear or Worry

Summary

Ideal body weight is important to good health. Although obtaining an ideal body weight is important, what is more important is maintaining that weight for life. Rapid weight loss often reflects a loss of muscle and water, not fat tissue, and can increase a person's risk for disease and obesity.

The gradual weight loss that results from a change in eating and exercise habits is more likely to be a permanent loss and one that is most beneficial to health. Social or group support, a realistic goal, a well-planned and individualized diet and exercise program, and a strong commitment to stick with it are important components of a successful weight loss and weight maintenance program.

References

1. Sande K, Mahan K: Nutrition care for weight management, in Krause M, Mahan L (eds): *Food, Nutrition, and Diet Therapy* ed 7. Philadelphia, WB Saunders Co, 1984, p 518.
2. Garn S, Clark D: Trends in fatness and origins in obesity, *Pediatrics,* 1976; 57:443-455.
3. Krause M, Mahan L: Balance and imbalance of body weight, in *Food, Nutrition, & Diet Therapy,* 6th ed. Philadelphia, WB Saunders, 1979, pp 553-577.
4. Greenwood M, Turkenkopf I: *Genetic and Metabolic Aspects, Obesity.* New York, Churchill Livingstone, 1983, pp 193-205.
5. Rona R: Social and family factors and obesity in children. *Ann Hum Bio* 1982; 9:131-45.
6. Hertzeler N: Obesity-impact on the family. *J Am Diet Assoc* 1981; 79:525-529.
7. Morris S: Feeding behaviors, food attitudes, and body fatness. *J Am Diet Assoc* 1982; 80:330-333.
8. Friedman R: What to tell patients about weight loss methods, Parts 1,2,3. *Post Med* 1982; 72:73-98.
9. Khoury P: Parent-offspring and sibling body mass index assessment. *Metabolism* 1983; 32:82.
10. Stunkard A: *Obesity.* Philadelphia, WB Saunders, 1980, pp 1-24.
11. Faust I: Nutrition and the fat cell. *Int J Obes* 1980; 4:314-21.
12. Swaminathan R: Thermic effect of feeding carbohydrate, fat, protein, and mixed meal in lean and obese subjects. *Am J Clin Nutr* 1985; 142:177.
13. Grossman S: The Neuroanatomy of eating and drinking behavior, in *Neuroendrocrinology.* Sunderland, Sinaier Assoc, Inc, 1980, pp 131-140.
14. Ibid, p 516.
15. Della Fera M, Baile C: Cholecystokinin octapeptide: Continuous picomole injections into the cerebral ventricles of sheep suppress feeding. *Science* 1979; 206:471.
16. Daniels J: The pathogenesis of obesity. *Psych Clin Nutr* 1985; 7:335-47.

17. Felig P: Insulin as the mediator of feeding related theromogensis. *Clin Phys* 1984; 4:267-73.
18. Morley J: Species differences in the response to cholecystokinin. *Ann NY Acad Sci* 1985; 448:413-416.
19. Bray G: Brown tissue and metabolic obesity. *Nutr Today* 1982; Jan/Feb:23-27.
20. Sacks P: Understanding obesity, Part I. *Nutr Rep* 1985; 3:52-53.
21. Sacks P: Understanding obesity, Part II. *Nutr Rep* 1985; 3:60-61.
22. Jung R, James W: Is obesity metabolic?, *Br J Hosp Med* 1980; 246:523-530.
23. Nair K: Thermic response to isoenergetic protein, carbohydrate, or fat meals in obese and lean subjects. *Clin Sci* 1983; 65:307-312.
24. Schwartz R: The thermic response to carbohydrate vs. fat feeding in man. *Metabolism* 1985; 34:85-93.
25. Bessard T: Energy expenditure and postparandial thermogenesis in obese women before and after weight loss. *Am J Clin Nutr* 1983; 38:680-693.
26. Griffith W: Food as a regulator of metabolism. *Am J Clin Nutr* 1965; 17:391-398.
27. Baily C: *Fit or Fat.* Boston, Houghton Mifflin Co, 1977, pp 1-56.
28. Bennett W: Dieting-ideology vs. physiology. *Psych Clin Nutr* 1984; 7:321-34.
29. Stillman I: *The Doctor's Quick Weight Loss Diet*, Englewood Cliffs, New Jersey, Prentice Hall Inc, 1968.
30. Atkins R: Dr. Atkins Diet Revolution. *The High Calorie Way To Stay Thin Forever.* New York, David McKay Inc Publishers, 1972.
31. Dietary Goals for the United States ed 2. *Select Committee on Nutrition and Human Needs,* United States Senate. Washington DC, US Government Printing Office, 1977, Publication No. 052-070-04376-8.
32. Geiselman P, Novin D: The role of carbohydrates in appetite, hunger, and obesity. *J Int Res* 1982; 3:203-223.
33. Wurtman J: Neurotransmitter control of carbohydrate consumption. *Ann NY Acad Sci* 1985; 443:145-151.

34. Wurtman R, Fernstom J: Control of brain monoamine synthesis by diet and plasma amino acids. *Am J Clin Nutr* 1975; 28:638-647.

35. Sande K, Mahan K: Nutritional care for weight management, in Krause M, Mahan L (eds): *Food, Nutrition, and Diet Therapy* ed 7. Philadelphia, WB Saunders Co, 1984, pp 520-521.

36. Clark R, Blackburn: Danger ahead? Fad diets for weight control. *The Professional Nutritionist* 1982; Summer:1-4.

37. *Weight Control Source Book*. Rosemont, Illinois, National Dairy Council, 1977, p 17.

38. Fisher M, Lachance P: Nutrition evaluation of published weight loss diets. *J Am Diet Assoc* 1985; 85:450-454.

39. *Recommended Dietary Allowances* ed 9. Committee on Dietary Allowances, Food and Nutrition Board, National Research Council. Washington DC, National Academy of Sciences, 1980, p 33.

40. Newton K: Weight management: Learning to self-regulate dietary habits. *Nutr Rep* 1986; 4:12-16.

41. Council on Foods and Nutrition: A critique of low-carbohydrate ketogenic weight reduction regimens: A review of Dr. Atkin's Revolution. Chicago, AMA Council on Foods and Nutrition. *JAMA* 1973; 224:10.

42. Rational of the diet-heart statement of the American Heart Association. *Arteriosclerosis* 1982; 4:177-191.

43. *Cancer Facts and Figures 1985*. American Cancer Society, National Headquarters, 90 Park Avenue, New York, NY, 10016.

44. *Healthy People, The Surgeon General's Report on Health Promotion and Disease Prevention,* US Dept. HEW, 1979, pp 50-62.

45. Block G, Dresser C, Hartmen A, et al: Nutrient sources in the American diet-quantitative data from the NHANES II survey: Macronutrients and fat. *Am J Epidem* 1985; 122:27-40.

46. Garrison R, Somer E: *The Nutrition Desk Reference.* New Canaan, Conn, Keats Publishing Co, 1985, pp 132-147.

47. Dietary levels of households in the United States, Spring 1965. *Agriculture Research Service,* US Department of Agriculture, 1968, pp 12-17.

48. *Ten State Nutrition Survey.* US Department of Health, Education, and Welfare, Health Series and Mental Health Administration Center for Disease Control. Atlanta GA, DHEW Publication No. (HMS) 72-8130-8134.

49. *First Health and Nutrition Examination Survey.* Public Health Service, Health Resources Administration, US Department of Health, 1971-1972.

50. Nationwide Food Consumption Survey, Spring 1980. Beltsville, MD, US Department of Agriculture, Science and Education Administration.

51. Dietary intake source data: United States 1976-1980. Data from the National Health Survey, Series 11, No. 231, DHHS Publication No. (PHS) 83-1681, March 1983.

52. Mertz W: Chromium: An essential nutrient. *Cont Nutr* 1982; 7:1-2.

53. Report of AHA Nutrition Committee: Rationale of the diet-heart statement of the American Heart Association. *Arteriosclerosis* 1982; 2:77.

54. American Cancer Society Special Report: *Nutrition and Cancer: Cause and prevention.* New York, American Cancer Society Inc, February 10, 1984.

55. Brewster L, Jacobsen M: *The Changing American Diet.* Washington DC, Center for Science in the Public Interest, 1983, p 47.

56. Leon G, The behavior modification approach to weight control. *Cont Nutr* 1979; 4:1-2

57. Ferguson J: *Habits Not Diets.* Palo Alto, CA, Bull Publishing, 1975, pp 1-2, 5-14.

58. Foreyt J: Limitations of behavioral treatment of obesity: Review and analysis. *J Behav Med* 1981; 4:159-173.

59. Kirshenbausm D: Behavioral treatment of adult obesity: Attentional Control and a 2 Year Follow-up. *Behav Res T* 1985; 23:675-682.

60. Bjorntorp P: Physiological and clinical aspects of exercise in obese persons. *Exer Sp Sci Rev* 1983; 11:159-180.

61. Brownell K, Stunkard A: Physical activity in the development of obesity, in Stunkard A (ed): *Obesity.* Philadelphia, WB Saunders Co, 1980 pp 300-324.
62. Brownell K, The Psychology and Physiology of Obesity. *J Am Diet Assoc* 1984; 84:406-14.
63. Hoerr S: Exercise: An alternative to fad diets for adolescent girls. *Phys Sports Med* 1984; 12:76-83.
64. Stern J: Diet and exercise, in Greenwood M (ed): *Obesity.* New York, Churchill Livingstone, 1983, pp 65-84.
65. Williams M: *Nutritional Aspects of Human Physical and Athletic Performance.* Springfield, Charles C. Thomas, 1976, pp 24-91.
66. Bielinsi R: Energy Metabolism During the Postexercise recovery in man. *Am J Clin N* 1985; 42:69-82.
67. Wasserthiel-Smoller S: Effective Dietary Intervention in hypertensives: Reducing the sodium and weight loss. *J Am Diet Assoc* 1985; 85:423-430.
68. Berchtold P: Epidemiology of obesity and hypertension. *Int J Obes* 1981; 5(Supp)1-7.
69. Exercise and Diabetes. *Nutr & MD,* 1984; 10:1-2.
70. Tremblay A: The reproducibility of a 3 day dietary recall. *Nut Res* 1983; 3:819-830.
71. Taylor K, Anthony L: *Clinical Nutrition,* New York, McGraw-Hill, 1983, pp 198-225.
72. Emery G: *Own Your Own Life.* New York, New American Library, 1982, pp 1-106.
73. *Recommended Dietary Allowances,* ed 9. Committee on Dietary Allowances, Food and Nutrition Board, Nutrition Research Council. Washington DC, National Academy of Sciences, 1980, pp 137-143.
74. Ibid, pp 1-39.
75. Nash J, Ormiston L: *Taking Charge of Your Weight and Well Being.* Palo Alto, CA, Bull Publishing, 1978, pp 381-473.
76. Van Itallie T: Obesity: Adverse effects on health and longevity. *Am J Clin Nutr* 1979; 32:2273.
77. *Heart Facts 1984.* Dallas, Texas, American Heart Association, National Center.
78. Gordon T, Kannel W: Obesity and cardiovascular disease: The Framingham study. *Clin Endocrinol Metabol* 1976; 5:367.

79. Stewart A: Effects of overweight. *Am J Pub Health.* 1983; 73:171-178.
80. Dustan H: Obesity and hypertension. *Ann Int Med* 1985; 103:1047-1049.
81. Crofford D: Report of the National Commission on Diabetes to the Congress of the United States (DHEW Publication Nol NIH 76-1018). Washington DC, US Government Printing Office, 1975.
82. Willett W, MacMahon B: Diet and cancer — An overview. *N Eng J Med* 1984; 310:697-703.
83. Howatson A, Carter D: High Fat-protein diet and pancreatic carcinogenesis. *Gut* 1983; 24:A985.
84. Rand C, Kuldau J: Stress and obesity. *Stress Med* 1985; 1:117-125.
85. Sande K, Mahan K: Nutritional care for weight management, in Krause M, Mahan L (eds): *Food, Nutrition, and Diet Therapy* ed 7. Philadelphia, WB Saunders Co, 1984, p 523.
86. Flack R, Grayer E: Consciousness-raising group for obese women. *Social Work* 1975; 20:484.
87. Bjorvell G: Personality traits in a group of severely obese patients. *Int J Obes* 1985; 9:257-266.
88. Wadden T, Stunkard J: Social and psychological consequences of obesity. *Ann Int Med* 1985; 103:1062-l067.

Glossary

Aerobic Exercise: Physical activity that involves large muscles of the legs or arms, that increases heart rate, and that is maintained continually for over 15 minues. Examples of aerobic exercise include walking, jogging, swimming, and bicycling.

Anaerobic Exercise: Physical activity that increases heart rate but is not continual movement. Examples of anaerobic exercise include weight lifting, volleyball, and football.

Atherosclerosis: The accumulation of fat deposits in the lining of the blood vessels. The arteries become roughened and narrowed and blood flow is restricted. Atherosclerosis is the underlying cause of heart attacks and stroke.

Basal Metabolic Rate (BMR): The amount of energy (calories) required to maintain basic body functions.

Brown Adipose Tissue (BAT): A type of fat that might maintain body temperature.

Carbohydrate: The starches and sugars in the diet.

Cardiovascular Disease: A disease of the heart and blood vessels often caused by the accumulation of fat in the arteries.

Cholecystokinine: A hormone that aids in digestion and might influence appetite.

Cervix: The opening to the uterus.

Colon: The large bowel located in the lower portion of the intestine.

Diabetes: A disorder in which the body's ability to use sugar is impaired because of inadequate production or utilization of the hormone insulin.

Endometrium: The lining of the uterus.

Enzymes: Proteins produced by the body that initiate and accelerate chemical reactions.

Estrogen: The female hormone that regulates the menstrual cycle and produces secondary sex characteristics.

Genetics: The heredity process whereby the characteristics of the body are passed from one generation to another.

Glucose: The building block of starch. Sugar. Blood sugar.

Hormone: A chemical substance produced by a group of cells or an organ, called an endocrine gland, that is released into the blood and transported to another organ or tissue, where it performs a specific action. Examples of hormones include estrogen, thyroxin, and insulin.

Hypertension: High blood pressure.

Hypothalamus: A portion of the brain that controls hunger, temperature regulation, water balance, and sleep.

Ideal Weight: A relationship between weight, height, and frame size determined to be the standard for normal.

Insulin: A hormone secreted by the pancreas that regulates blood sugar.

Ketosis: A state where incomplete breakdown products of fat metabolism called ketones are present in the blood.

Metabolism: The sum total of all body processes, whereby the body converts foods into tissues, breaks down and repairs tissues, and converts complex substances into simple ones for energy.

Morbid Obesity: Body weight greater than 30% above ideal as fat tissue.

Obesity: A body weight that exceeds 20% of the ideal as fat tissue.

Osteoarthritis: A degeneration of the joints that results in joint deformity and pain.

Overweight: Between 10% and 20% above normal weight according to the Height-Weight Table. The excess weight is fat weight.

Pancreas: The organ responsible for the production and secretion of numerous digestive enzymes and the hormone insulin responsible for the regulation of blood sugar (glucose).

Pituitary Gland: An endocrine gland located in the brain that regulates the growth of all tissues, the hormonal activity of the sex organs, and blood pressure.

Prostate: Gland located at the beginning of the urethera in males that secretes a fluid that nourishes and aids in the transport of seminal fluid.

Serotonin: A hormone-like substance produced in the brain that regulates mood and sleep.

Thermogenesis: The production of body heat.

Triglycerides: One of the three classes of fats; common name is fat or oil.

Thyroxin: The hormone produced by the thyroid gland that regulates metabolism.

Tryptophan: An amino acid that is the building block of serotonin.

Index

Notes